Alkaline Diet for Beginners

Understand PH, Eat Well and Reclaim Your Health with Easy Alkaline Diet Recipes.

Tamara White

ISBN: 9781731259899

Alkaline Blended Juice

Coated Sprout Salad

Mashed Kale Chickpea

SMOOTHIE RECIPES

Jive Green Lentil Smoothie

Smooth Alkaline Super Green Shake

Cucumber Soy Shake with Coconut

Green Power Cocktail

Alkaline Blackberry Smoothie

Seasonal Greens Smoothie

Mixed Cucumber Smoothie

Fine Herbs With Green Smoothie

Green Biggie Smoothie

Mixed Berry Smoothie

MAIN DISH

Alkaline Roasted Broccoli

Easy Alfredo Alkaline Pasta

Mashed Cauliflower Potatoes

Quinoa With Lemon And Apple

Quinoa Sweet Potato With Carrot

Zucchini Spinach With Lemon Pesto

Avocado Papaya Arugula Salad

Mixed Vegetables With Pumpkin Dressing

Vanilla Quinoa Porridge

Spiced-up Sprouted Stir-Fry

Vegetables Roast

Avocado-Adzuki Bean Stuffed Lettuce Cups

Easy Alkaline Risotto

Alkaline Cauliflower Rice With Vegetable Curry (Anti-Cancer)

Haricots Verts With Herbs And Shallots

Special Season Broccoli Brussels Sprouts

Spaghetti Squash Quinoa Stuffed

Roasted Cauliflower And Coriander, Turmeric with Mint

Broccoli with Cashew Cream Salad

Artichoke & Kale, Hemp Pesto

SNACKS RECIPES

Cucumber Bites with Tuna Mix

Apple Collard Coconut vinegar Wrap

Alkaline Tasty Raw Chili

California Chia Pudding

Alkaline Tasty Jalapenos Poppers

Tuna And Kale Stuffed Avocado

Alkaline Mashed Avocado Wraps

Alkaline Pumpkin Fries

Gallant Grilled Veggies

Alkaline Kohlrabi Carrot

Alkalizing Green Pasta

Winter Indoor Timely Pasta

Perfect Marinated Zucchini Squash

SOUP RECIPES

Creamy Citrus- Cilantro Dressing

Spinach Broccoli And Ginger Soup

Kale Soup With Creamy Red Lentil

Chilled Avocado, Watercress Soup

Curry Powder Carrot Soup

Healthy Healing Soup

Broccoli-Creamy Avocado Soup

Fresh Harvest Vegetable Soup

White Bean With Pumpkin And Sage Soup

Cauliflower-Swiss Emmenthal-Soup

Greek Lentils Flaky Soup

Easy Alkaline Porridge

Cucumber- Avocado Sushi Rolls

SALADS RECIPES

Avocado Cole Slaw Dressing

Avocado Apple Sesame Salad

Healthy Brussels Sprouts

Healthy Fresh Vegetable Salad

Tofu Broccoli Salad

Carrot-Fennel With Pomegranate Salad

Alkaline Almond Celery- Salad

Alkaline Special Salad

Alkaline Intercontinental Salad

Avocado Wild Garlic Salad

DESSERT

Alkaline Avocado Chocolate

Alkaline Raw Chocolate Pudding

Alkaline Luxury Figs

Pineapple Slaw With Kale

Almond with Macademia- Fresh Cherries

Alkaline Avocado Tomato Soup

Quinoa Mango Salad With Asparagus And Nuts

INTRODUCTION

What really is Alkaline Diet?

An alkaline diet — also called the alkaline acid diet, alkaline ash diet, acid alkaline diet, acid ash diet, and also called the pH diet — it assist in balancing the PH level of blood concerning the body fluids, including your urine and blood. Your pH is determined partially by the gravity of mineral properties of foods you eat. Every life forms and living organism rely on maintaining a proper pH levels, as the saying goes that there cannot be disorder and disease in a body with balanced PH.

The concept of acid ash assumption assist in making up the alkaline diet precept. Regarding research by Bone and Mineral expert, "The hypothesis of the acid-ash insinuates that grain and protein foods, having little potassium, generates a net acid excretion (NAE), let out calcium from the skeleton, generates more urine calcium, and diet acid load, which leads to osteoporosis.

The aim of the alkaline diet is the prevention of this kind of happening through consideration food pH levels, an effort to reduce dietary acid intake. Although this statement is not widely accepted by some experts, more than half all recognize that it is required by human life to have a tight regulated blood pH level of about 7.365 to 7.4.
Your pH can stay with the range of 7.35 to 7.45, it all depends on your diet, what you ate last, what time it is and time you went to the bathroom last.

What exactly is the meaning of "pH level"?

Potential of hydrogen (pH).This is a way of measuring acidity and alkalinity in the body. A measurement done on a scale of 0 to 14. If a solution is high in acidic, then the lower in PH. A higher alkaline, will result in a higher number. A PH of 7.4 is considered healthy, a PH of 7 is regarded as neutral, though PH levels are not all

the same throughout the entire body, with the most acidic region being the
stomach.

Any small alteration in the pH level of any organisms can pose a real challenge. For
instance, as a result of increase deposition in the Carbon dioxide, the ocean' PH has
reduced from 8.2 to 8.1 which is greatly affecting various ocean life forms. The pH
level is very important to grow plants, hereby affecting the mineral composition of
the foods we eat.
 Minerals in the human body, soil and ocean, are used as enhancer to maintain
maximum pH levels, so a rise in acidity, results in a fall in minerals.

Testing Your PH for Alkaline Balance

Our major focus here is pH of your saliva, urine, and blood. Your blood must be
tightly regulated at a constant pH of 7.365 and never changes.

Note: The purpose of this is not because you want to change your blood PH. When
you test saliva or urine, the PH you get is for the fluid that your body eliminate and
not the PH of your internal environment. Its needful that your body maintains a
narrow range of PH of 7.365-7.45.Although there might be differences between the
range you find in your saliva and urine as the body discharges plenty acids, which is
a good thing for maintaining your internal PH. It might be more convenient to test
your saliva than urine but urine reflects a better process of what the body undergo
to eliminate acid from the body.

Saliva and Urine PH Testing

It's a very easy process testing your PH, at least it a good way to boost motivation
and track your progress.
The saliva
Your saliva PH range is expected to be between 7.0 and 7.5
How to test Saliva PH:
Its best immediately you wake up in the morning before anything else or you can
wait two hours after teeth brushing of food. Start by holding saliva in your mouth,
swallow it and repeat a few times just to be certain your saliva is clean. Afterwards
place some of the spit on a PH stip. A chart will be provided at the back of the kit,
different shades of color reflects alkaline or acid state. Jot down the date, time and
number to keep track of your progress.

How to test Urine PH

It shows the working performance of the body towards maintaining a proper PH blood. It reflects the body's effort, through the kidneys, lungs and adrenals in regulating PH by excretion of acids, and minerals like, sodium, calcium, potassium. Your urine PH range is expected to be between 6.5 and 7.5. A Ph of below 6.5 may indicate a system overwhelming.

This is also similar to the way you carry out your saliva test. Its best immediately you wake up in the morning you can urinate directly into a container and insert the PH strips or urinate on the Strip directly. A chart will be provided at the back of the kit, different shades of color reflects alkaline or acid state. Jot down the date, time and number to keep track of your progress.

How an Alkaline Diet works

Tips on how alkaline diets can be beneficial:

Because of the ratio of potassium to sodium in most people's diets which has dramatically changed, people consume now more sodium as potassium which are low in essential vitamins, antioxidants, fiber, magnesium and potassium. What most people consume now is simple sugars, refined fats, sodium and chloride. This has caused an increase in "metabolic acidosis" simply put, so many people PH level is low. The danger this pose is gradual loss of organ functions, it cause rapid aging, degenerates tissue, it cause the cells, bone, tissue and organs to loose important minerals.

Signs You've Got an Unhealthy Gut

Digestive discomfort, diahorrea, gas, and Bloating
Frequent feelings of anxiety
Inability to focus, lack of concentration and Poor memory
Depressive thoughts or ongoing depression
A short irritability/fuse and mood swings
Pre-diabetes or symptoms of Diabetes
Allergies
Already diagnosed autoimmune disease
Frequent use of antibiotics, or frequent infections
Topical skin complaints such as rosacea, eczema

Alkaline Diet Benefits

1. Protects Muscle Mass and Bone Density

Minerals is very important in maintaining and developing bone structure. The more alkalizing vegetables and fruits you eats, you stand a better chance at protecting yourself against muscle wasting as you age and decreasing bone strength "sarcopenia".
Following alkaline diet will help maintain minerals ratios crucial to maintaining lean muscle mass and build bones, including phosphate, magnesium and calcium, increase generation of vitamin D absorption and growth hormones, a way to protects bones and reduce plenty chronic diseases.

2. Help to Maintain a Healthy Weight

Increased eating of alkaline-forming foods and reducing the eating of acid-forming foods has been proven to prevent the body from obesity, it decrease inflammation and leptin levels, also affects fat-burning abilities and your hunger.

3. Protects Against Cancer and Helps Boost Immune Function

Lack of necessary minerals by the cells to fully oxygenate the body fully or dispose of waste, is dangerous to the body. Mineral loss will reduce vitamin absorption, pathogens and toxins will be accumulated in the body which damage the immune system.

4. Lowers Chronic Pain and Inflammation

Research has showed that there is a connection with alkaline diet and reduction in chronic pain.

5. Reduce Risk of Stroke and Hypertension

Alkaline diet performs an anti-aging effects on your body, is helps to push up growth of hormone production and decreases inflammation. It helps boost cardiovascular health and protect against issues like memory loss, stroke, kidney stones, hypertension and high cholesterol.

6. Kick against Magnesium Deficiency and Improve Vitamin Absorption

For the efficient functioning of volume of bodily processes and enzyme systems, an increase in magnesium is necessary. A lot of people are magnesium deficient, which can translate to anxiety, sleep troubles, headaches, muscle pains and heart complications. Presence of magnesium is needed to boost vitamin D and avert vitamin D shortage, essential to endocrine functioning and overall immune.

List of Acid and Base Foods

In order for the human body to function properly, it's necessary to maintain equilibrium, or homeostasis. To perform this, partly by maintaining pH, a way of measuring acidity and alkalinity in the body, also referred to as acid-base balance. To maintain the acid-base balance, what you eat plays a basic role. According to the research, a healthy diet is two-thirds base foods and one-third acid foods

Fruits and Vegetables

A lot of vegetables and fruits falls under base foods, to break it down, when foods like these are consumed, they effect the alkalinity in your body. Some food are more alkaline than others. For instance kale and celery are more alkaline than mushrooms, and bananas and onions are more alkaline than watermelon. But peas and lentils are the exemption, have an acidic effect on the body.

Grains and Grain Products

Grains in general and any grain made food have an acidic effect on the body. Pasta, refined bread and whole-meal, brown and white rice, rye, oats, millet buckwheat, spelt and amaranth.

Seafood and Meat

All animal flesh in general have an acidic effect on the body. From steak to salmon, and most acidic flesh are processed meats (canned corned beef) rabbit, goose, trout, prawns, sardines, liver, and shellfish.

Dairy and Eggs

Any products made from milk and Milk in general are acidic, with a few exceptions like, cottage cheese, processed cheese, Camembert, Edam, reduced-fat and whole milk and Parmesan.
Eggs are also acidic, but the whites are not as acidic as the yolks.

Full-fat Kefir cheese is neutral, i.e. neither an acidic nor base effect on the body. Whey is base food.

Fats and oils vary
Sunflower seed and olive oils are neutral (you already understand the meaning of neutral with full fat kefir cheese)
Margarine is base, Butter is acidic.
With the exception of hazelnuts, which are base, most nuts are acidic. Sweets also run the gamut and honey and brown sugar are base, white sugar is neutral.
Ice cream with fruit is base but vanilla ice cream is acidic.
Vinegars and herbs and are all base foods.

Beverage Choices
Most fruit juices are base. White and red wines, coffee, vegetable juices, mineral water, cocoa, and Tea, are all base. Beer vary, draft and stout and beers are base. Pale ale is acidic, Sugary sodas are acidic.

Alkaline water
What is alkaline water?
What exactly do you understand by alkaline water? Some people believe it can help prevent chronic diseases, slow aging process, and regulate body's pH level.

Alkaline water is water that rich in alkalizing compounds, including bicarbonate, magnesium, potassium, silica, and calcium. Alkaline water has a higher pH level of 9 to 11 and also has less acidic than regular drinking water. It is believe that alkaline water can and help your body metabolize nutrients more effectively and also neutralize the acid in your bloodstream, leading to optimum health.

Benefits Of Alkaline Water
Helps prevent cancer
Weight loss
Detoxifying, skin health and hydration
Immune system support
Colon-cleansing properties
Anti-aging properties
.

Food to make your Body Alkaline
A further breaking down of the list:

Alkaline Forming Foods
Flaxseed Oil
Olive Oil
Coconut Oil
Almonds
Chia Seeds
Quinoa
Ginger
Turmeric
Garlic
Capsicum (Bell Pepper)
Sweet Potato
Squash
Pumpkin
Asparagus
Artichoke
Grapefruit
Limes
Lemons
Rocket (Arugula)
Chives
Cabbage
Broccoli
Watercress
Lentils
Chickpeas (Garbanzo)
Green Beans
Collards
Siverbeet (Chard)
Kale (all varieties)
Spring Onions (Scallions/Salad Onions)
Basil
Celery
Cucumber
Beets
Coriander/Cilantro
Lettuce (all varieties)
Spinach
Avocado and heaps, the list could go on...

Acidic Forming Foods
Pasta
Crisps
Cookies
Baked Goods (muffins etc)
Pastries
Jams
Sweets
Caffeine
Alcohol
Fruits (eeek, see below)
Spelt
Wheat
Dairy
Excessive Animal Protein
Processed Meats (esp. bacon)
Processed Foods
Fast Food
Takeaway
Trans-Fats
Deep Fried Foods
Chips
Pizza
Chocolate
All sugar (including syrups)

Some of the habits that can cause acidity in your body

Shallow breathing
Processed and refined foods
Poor eating and chewing habits
Pollution
Pesticides and herbicides
Over-exercise
Food coloring and preservatives

Chemicals Exposure and radiation from microwaves, cell phones, computers, building materials and household cleansers
Excess hormones from beauty products, foods, and health, and plastics
Excess non-grass-fed sources animal meats in the diet
Lack of exercise
Low levels of fiber in the diet
Decreasing level of nutrient in foods because of industrial farming
Chronic stress
Artificial sweeteners
Antibiotic overuse
High caffeine intake
Alcohol and drug use

BREAKFAST

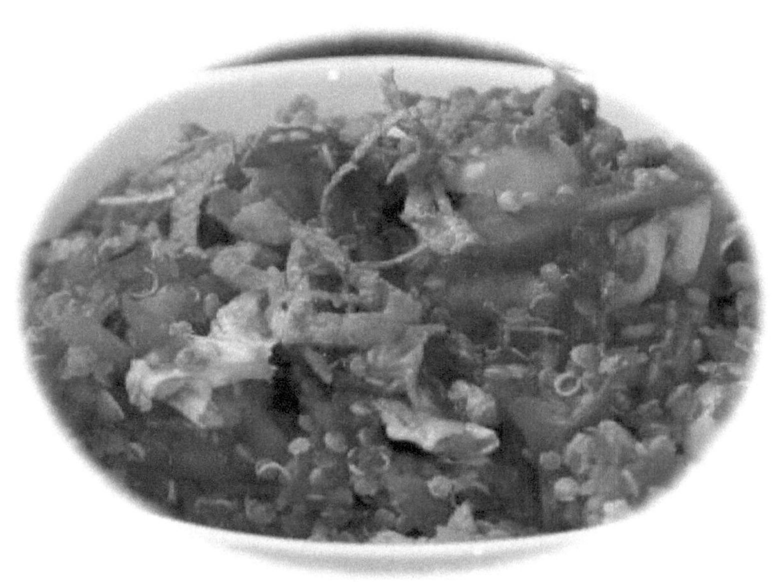

Toasted Sprouted Bread Avocado

Servings: 2

Ingredients:

1 teaspoon of olive oil

1 cup Cherry tomatoes

1 avocado, roughly mashed

2 slice sprouted bread, toasted

Parsley and Sea salt, to Seasoning

Preparations:

1. Spread mashed avocado on bread.

2. Add the cherry tomatoes on one side, drizzled with olive oil, season with parsley and Sea salt.

Friendly Quinoa Bowl

Servings: 2

Ingredients:

4 tablespoon of soaked almonds

2 teaspoon of olive oil

2 cup of cooked broccoli

1 cup of cooked quinoa

Coriander, parsley and Sea salt to Seasoning

Preparations:

1. In a bow, add all the ingredients. Enjoy!

Simple Chia Seed Pudding

Servings: 2

Ingredients:

1 tablespoon of honey

½ cup of berries

2 cup vanilla almond milk, unsweetened (or coconut milk)

½ cup of chia seeds

Preparations:

1. Mix honey, chia seeds and coconut milk or almond in small glass. Place in the fridge overnight to set.

2. It should be thick by morning and the chia seeds have gelled. Remove and top with berries. Enjoy!

Servings: 1

Ingredients:

1 cup of unsweetened almond milk

1 tablespoon of flaxseeds

1 tablespoon of chia seeds

¼ cup of raw pumpkin seeds

¼ cup of raw almonds

Cinnamon and stevia to taste

Preparations:

1. Place all ingredients in a bowl, season with cinnamon and stevia to taste.

2. Allow to soak overnight. Enjoy your tasty breakfast in the morning!

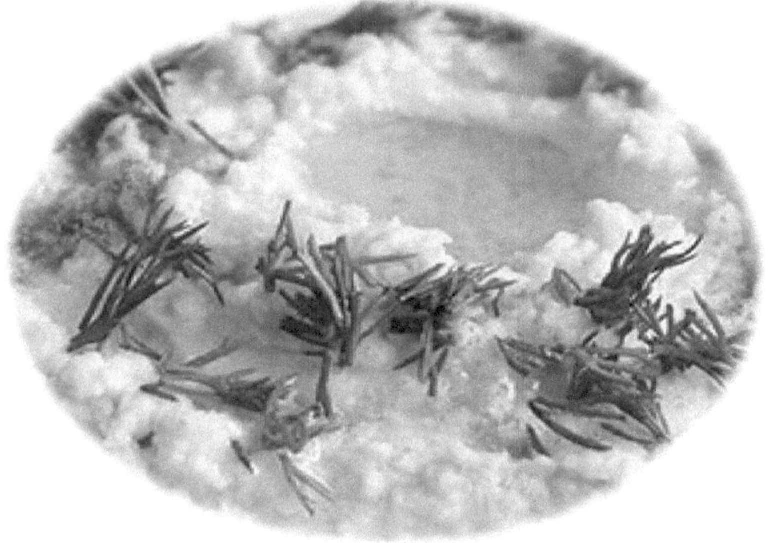

Easy Breakfast Marinated Mushrooms

Servings: 1

Ingredients:

A few drops of sesame oil

Pinch of chopped black pepper

Pinch of Himalayan salt

Pinch of chopped rosemary

Pinch of chopped spring onion

1 tablespoon of Balsamic vinegar

½ dozen of thinly sliced mushrooms

Preparations:

1. Combine all ingredients in a bowl. Place in the fridge overnight to set.

2. Serve with your favorite salad and enjoy.

Quinoa Breakfast Burrito Dish

Prep time: 10 mins

Cook time: 35 mins

Serving: 2

Ingredients:

Handful of chopped cilantro

2 sliced avocados

1 teaspoon cumin

4 minced cloves garlic

2 freshly juiced limes

4 green sliced onions

2 15-oz cans of adzuki beans, rinsed and drained

2 cups of filtered water

1 cup of quinoa

Preparations:

1. Add the water in a pot and cook the quinoa over high heat.

2. Cover and reduce heat to low immediately the water comes to a boil, cook for 15-20 minutes or until quinoa is cooked and water is absorbed.

3. Meanwhile, cook beans on low heat in a small saucepan. Stir cumin, garlic, lime juice, and onions, cook for 10 to 15 minutes.

4. Serve quinoa into different serving bowls, top with cilantro, beans and avocado. Enjoy!

Pistachios, Brussels Sprouts and Lemon

Prep time: 5 mins

Cook time: 6 mins

Serving: 4

Ingredients:

16 large Brussels sprouts, core and leaves separated. Cut sprout end off and also peel leaves off

1 lemon juice and Zest

¾ cup of shelled pistachios

2 tablespoons of olive oil, extra virgin

Pepper to taste

Salt to taste

Preparations:

1. In a large skillet, heat olive oil over medium-high heat. Sauté lemon zest and pistachios for 1 minute.

2. Add Brussels leaves, cook and toss about 5 minutes until crisp and still bright green. Add lemon juice and season with salt and pepper. Enjoy!

Early Sunrise Muesli Recipe

Servings: 1

Ingredients:

Dash of cinnamon

½ cup of apple, chopped (optional)

1 tablespoon of almond, sliced (optional)

1 cup of almond or coconut milk, unsweetened (from a carton)

½ cup of gluten free rolled oats

Preparations:

1. Combine all ingredients in a bowl. Place in the fridge overnight. A lovely breakfast cereal for you in the morning. You can also warm it in the morning if you want it hot.

Option #2: cook the oats and add in your fruit and nuts.

Morning Avocado Salad

Servings: 1
Ingredients:
Half a lemon juice
Half a red onion, chopped
2 tomatoes, chopped
One spoon of chili sauce
4 handfuls of baby spinach
A handful of chopped almonds
1 pink chopped grapefruit
1 Avocado, chopped
Half a pack of firm tofu, chopped
2 Tortillas
Preparations:
1. Heat the tortillas in the oven for 8 to 10 minutes.
2. Combine tomatoes, tofu and onions with some chilli sauce in a bowl, place inside the refrigerator to cool.
3. Add the avocado, grapefruit and almonds. Mix everything together and place into the bowl.
4. Top with a Squeeze of fresh lemon juice!

Alkaline Blended Juice

Prep time: 10 mins
Cook time: 1 mins
Servings: 2
Ingredients:
1 cup ice cubes, plus more if needed
1/4 tsp of Celtic sea salt
1 tsp of balsamic vinegar
1/3 (17g) cup of packed basil leaves
1 small lemon, peeled and seeded
1 medium tomato, slice
1 medium red bell pepper, topped and seeded
2 (270g) cups of fresh strawberries, firmly packed
2 (330g) cups of diced fresh watermelon
Optional boosters:
1/8 tsp of red pepper flakes
2 tbsp of goji berries

1/4 (30g) cup raw frozen cauliflower
Preparations:
1. Combine all the ingredients into the blender and blend for 30 seconds to 1 minutes on high until smooth.

Coated Sprout Salad

Prep time: 5 mins
Servings: 1
Ingredients:
Black pepper
Fresh juice of a lemon
1 tsp of coconut oil
A handful of chopped parsley
1 diced spring onion
1 chopped cucumber
Celtic sea salt
50 gms of sprouts
Preparations:
1. Add parsley, pepper, salt and lemon juice to make dressing. Add cucumber and spring onion, mix.
2. Rinse the sprouts and stir into the dressing. Serve immediately.

Mashed Kale Chickpea

Prep time: 5 minutes
Cook time: 20 minutes
Servings: 1-2
Ingredients:
2 tbs of coconut oil
400 gms of chickpeas
A bunch of kale
1 chopped shallot
3 tbs of minced garlic
Celtic sea salt for taste
Preparations:
1. Add olive oil in a saucepan, fry the chopped shallot and minced garlic, heat until its golden brown. Add some, garlic, onion and kale.
Add chick peas 6 minutes before the end of cooking. Season with sea salt and stir.

SMOOTHIE RECIPES

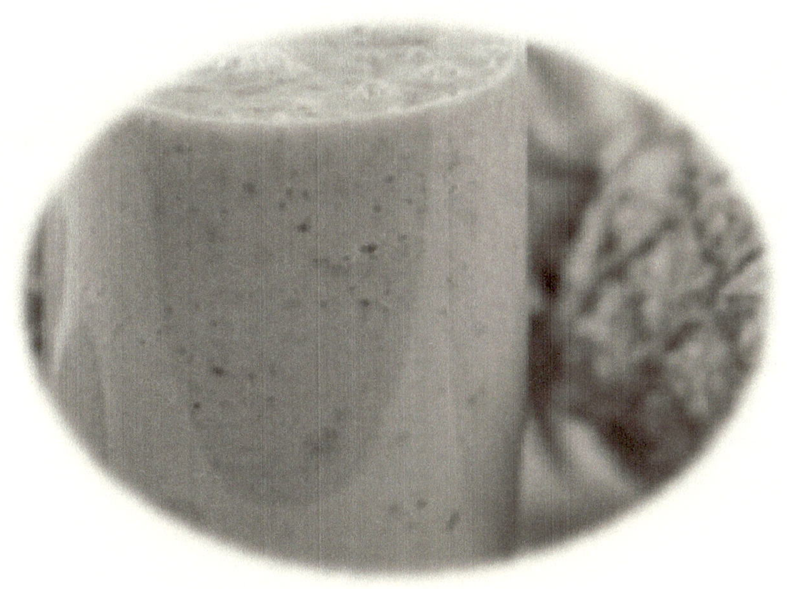

Jive Green Lentil Smoothie

Prep time: 5
Servings: 6
Ingredients:
1/2 chopped cucumber
1 cup of chopped Kale, spines removed
3/4 cup red Lentils, cooked
1 medium cored and chopped Apple
1 medium Banana
1/2 cup chilled Water (preferably alkaline water)
3/4 cup Ice cubes crushed (preferably alkaline water)
1/2 cup of Greek yogurt, vanilla, fat-free
3 tablespoon of Honey
3 tablespoon of Lemon juice
1/2 tablespoon of Spirulina, dried
Preparations:
1. Combine all the ingredients in a blender blend until smooth.

Smooth Alkaline Super Green Shake

Serving: 1-2
Ingredients:
Water (preferably alkaline water)
Cubes of ice, best made with alkaline water
1 tablespoon of SuperGreens Powder
1 peeled lime
1 cup of fresh spinach leaves
1 cup of cabbage
½ medium cucumber
1 avocado
Preparations:
1. With the exception of ice cubes and SuperGreens, combine all ingredients into blender, blend until smooth.
2 Serve on ice in a glass and add water as desired.

Cucumber Soy Shake with Coconut

Serving: 1

Ingredients:

7 cubes of ice (best made with alkaline water)

1 teaspoon of organic vanilla

 2 small shredded cucumbers

50ml fresh unsweetened coconut milk, 500ml

Fresh unsweetened soy milk, 500ml

Preparations:

1. Combine all the ingredients in a blender blend until smooth in less 1 minute.

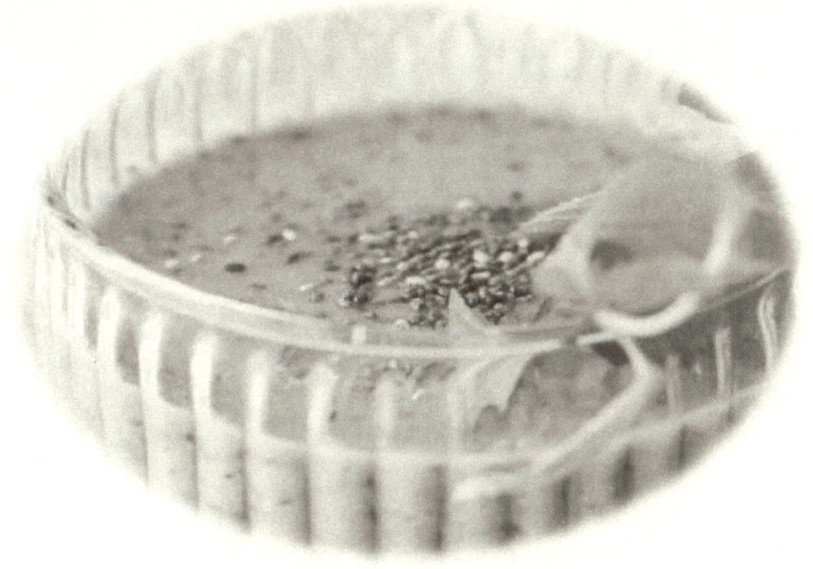

Green Power Cocktail

Serving: 2 shakes

Ingredients:

½ cup of Wheat Grass

1 cup of Beets

1 cup of Kale

4 cups of Green Tops

4 cups of Sprouts

Preparations:

1. Use a juicer to extract all ingredients and enjoy cold or warm.

Alkaline Blackberry Smoothie

Serving: 2

Ingredients:

½ teaspoon of vanilla

2 tablespoon of coconut oil

1 fresh lime juiced

1 large of bunch of kale

½ cup of frozen strawberries

1 cup of frozen blackberries

1 ½ cups of almond or coconut milk, unsweetened

1 tablespoon of raw almond butter (Optional)

Preparations:

1. Start by blending the coconut milk and kale first, then pour in the rest ingredients, and blend until you have a smooth mixture.

Seasonal Greens Smoothie

Prep time: 5 minutes

Serving: 1

Ingredients:

1 tablespoon of coconut oil

Dash of cinnamon

1 chopped pear, preferably frozen

½ banana, preferably frozen

1 large handful of spinach

1 cup of coconut water

1 tablespoon of chia seeds (optional)

Preparations:

1. Combine all the ingredients in a blender blend until smooth

Mixed Cucumber Smoothie

Prep time: 5 mins

Servings: 2

Ingredients:

1 cup Ice cubes, use alkaline water

1 1/2 cup of alkaline Water

3 drop of Stevia sweetener

2 tablespoon of fresh Lime juice

1/2 medium Jalapeno pepper (stemmed, seeded, de-ribbed)

1/8 Cucumber, peeled

1 medium stalk of Celery

Preparations:

1. Combine all the ingredients in a blender blend until you have a smooth mixture.

Fine Herbs With Green Smoothie

Prep time: 5 mins

Servings: 1

Ingredients:

1/2 teaspoon of Chia seeds, ground (optional)

1 whole fresh Lime juice

1 cup of Water

1 1/2 tsp minced Ginger root (optional)

1/4 cup of diced Pineapple, banana or mango

1 medium Pear

2 medium Celery stalk

1/2 cup of Cucumber

1/2 cup of Cilantro (coriander)

1/2 cup of Kale

Preparations:

1. Combine all ingredients in a blender and blend until you have smooth mixture.

Green Biggie Smoothie

Prep time: 10

Servings: 1

Ingredients:

1/4 cup of Water, alkaline

1 cup of Spinach

1 cup of diced Pineapple

1/2 cup of sliced Mango

1 cup of Kale, stems removed

1 cup of Ice cubes

1/2 Avocado

1 medium Apple

Preparations:

1. Combine all ingredients in a blender and blend, increasing the speed slowly until you have smooth mixture. Enjoy!

Mixed Berry Smoothie

Servings: 1

Ingredients:

1 cup of coconut water

1 tablespoon of chia seeds

1 tablespoon of coconut oil

1 teaspoon of cinnamon

1 lime, freshly squeezed

1/2 frozen banana

½ cup of mixed frozen berries

1 large handful spinach

Preparations:

1. Combine all ingredients in a blender and blend until you have smooth mixture.

MAIN DISH

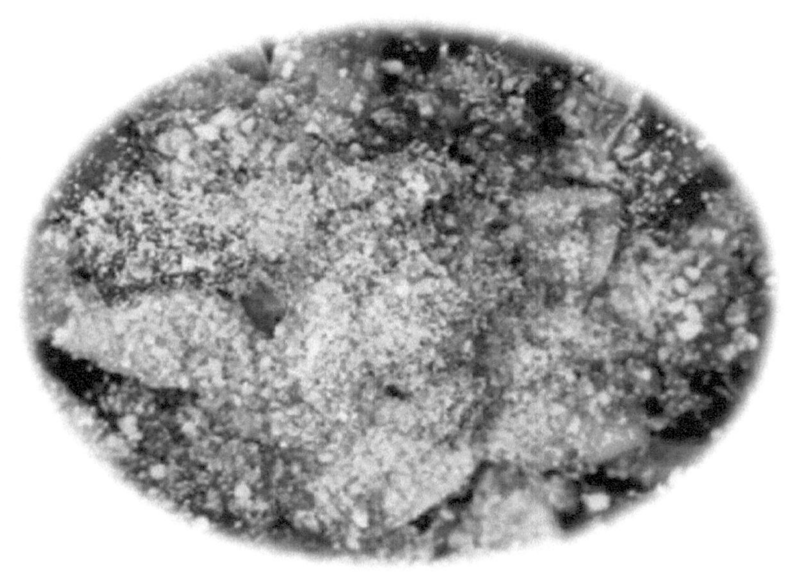

Alkaline Roasted Broccoli

Prep time: 5 mins
Cook time: 30 mins
Serving: 4
Ingredients:
Black pepper to taste
10 fresh garlic cloves, sliced
3 tablespoon of extra virgin olive oil
Sea salt to taste
1 large bunch broccoli florets, cut into bite size pieces
Preparations:
1. Preheat oven to 450 F.
2. Arrange the broccoli and garlic in a bowl, Add olive oil, pepper and salt. Stir well to coat
3. Spread evenly on a baking sheet and Roast about 10 minutes, then flip and roast for extra 10 to 20 minutes, or as you desired crispiness. Serve and enjoy!

Easy Alfredo Alkaline Pasta

Prep time: 3 mins
Cook time: 4 mins
Serving: 4
Ingredients:
Alfredo Cauliflower Sauce:
1/4 teaspoon of smoked or regular paprika
1 teaspoon of fresh squeezed lemon juice
1 cup of almond
1/3 cup of yeast free vegetable broth
1 15 ounce can of white beans, rinsed and drained
Sea salt to taste
2 tablespoon of extra virgin olive oil
1 finely chopped clove garlic
1 (about 1.5 cups) sliced yellow onion
1 roughly chopped head cauliflower
Black pepper
Noodles:
12 sun-dried thinly sliced tomatoes
8 cups of baby spinach
1/4 cup of filtered water

1/2 tablespoon of coconut oil

2-4 zucchinis, spiralized

Preparations:

Alfredo Cauliflower Sauce:

1. Heat up the oven to 400F.

2. Mix the garlic, yellow onion, and chopped cauliflower together in a large bowl. Add extra virgin olive oil and a generously sprinkle of sea salt, toss to coat.

3. Set on a baking sheet in a single layer and roast for 45 to 60 minutes at 400F, or until soft. Remove from the oven carefully.

4. Combine the mixture, smoked paprika, lemon juice, almond, vegetable broth, white beans, and black pepper to a blender. Blend until creamy and smooth. Add more broth or milk to adjust the consistency, if needed. Season to taste then set aside.

For Noodles:

5. In a large sauté pan, heat coconut oil, Cook and stir the zucchini noodles, black pepper and sea salt, until noodles are soft, about 3 to 5 minutes. Set aside.

6. Bring 1/4 cup of water to boil over medium-heat in a large saucepan. Add spinach and cook and stir about 1 to 2 minutes or until it is wilted. Mix in the sun-dried tomatoes, add the Alfredo cauliflower sauce earlier set aside, and toss in zucchini noodle. Enjoy!

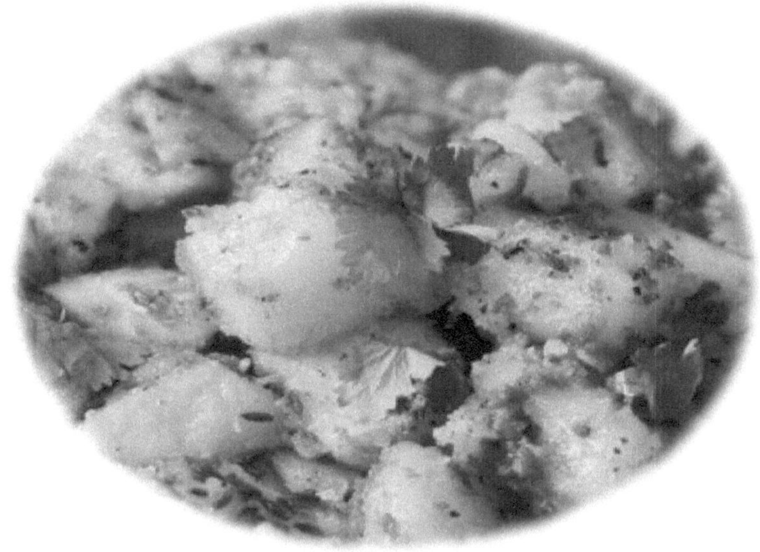

Mashed Cauliflower Potatoes

Prep time: 10 mins

Cook time: 15 mins

Serving: 4

Ingredients:

2 teaspoon of chopped parsley

2 teaspoon of coconut oil

1 teaspoon of garlic powder

1 carrot

1/4 cup of yeast free vegetable broth

1 chopped head of cauliflower

1 chopped onion

3 minced cloves garlic

2 teaspoon of chopped rosemary

Sea salt

Black pepper to taste

Preparations:

1. In a large pot, heat the coconut oil, sauté garlic and onion until slightly browned, about 5 minutes.

2. Add in vegetable broth, carrot, and cauliflower. Cook until heated through, then simmer for 10 minutes on medium-low. Add more of the vegetable broth if needed.

3. Add parsley, rosemary, salt, garlic powder and pepper. Mash using either an immersion blender, food processor or a blender until smooth. Enjoy!

Quinoa With Lemon And Apple

Prep time: 10 mins

Cook time: 25 mins

Serving: 2

Ingredients:

Cinnamon

½ lemon

1 apple

½ cup of quinoa, rinse and drained

Preparations:

1. Add the water in a pot and cook the quinoa over high heat.

2. Cover and reduce heat to low immediately the water comes to a boil, cook for 15-20 minutes or until quinoa is cooked and water is absorbed.

3. Grate in the apple and cook for 1/2 minutes, squeeze a little lemon and grate in lemon zest to taste.

4. Transfer into individual bowls and sprinkle with cinnamon.

Quinoa Sweet Potato With Carrot

Prep time: 3 mins

Cook time: 15-20 mins

Serving: 4

Ingredients:

¼ cup of extra virgin olive oil

1 lemon juice and Zest

½ cup of almond slivers

1 large bunch of sage, (cut into ribbons)

1 grated carrot

1 grated beet

1 grated sweet potato

1 15-oz can of white beans

½ bunch of Swiss chard, (cut into ribbons)

2 chopped shallots

4 minced garlic cloves

4 cups of vegetable broth

Sea salt

Black pepper

2 cups of quinoa, rinsed, soaked for 20 minutes

Preparations:

1. Cook shallots, garlic, vegetable broth, and quinoa on medium heat for 15 to 20 minutes in a pot or until liquid is absorbed. Stir in the remaining ingredients and cook until heated through. Enjoy!

Zucchini Spinach With Lemon Pesto

Prep time: 8 mins

Cook time: 5 mins

Serving: 4

Ingredients:

1⁄2 cup of cherry tomatoes sliced in half

1⁄2 cup of extra virgin olive oil

1⁄4 cup of cashews

1 small to medium lemon Juice

3 minced garlic cloves

1⁄4 cup of basil

3 cups of baby spinach

4 zucchinis, spiralized

Salt and Pepper to taste

Preparations:

1. Pulse cashews, garlic, basil, and spinach in a food processor until chopped finely. Then slowly add lemon juice and olive oil with food processor still running. Season with salt and pepper.

2. Combine the spinach Lemon Pesto and zucchini pasta in a serving bowl. Garnish with sliced cherry tomatoes.

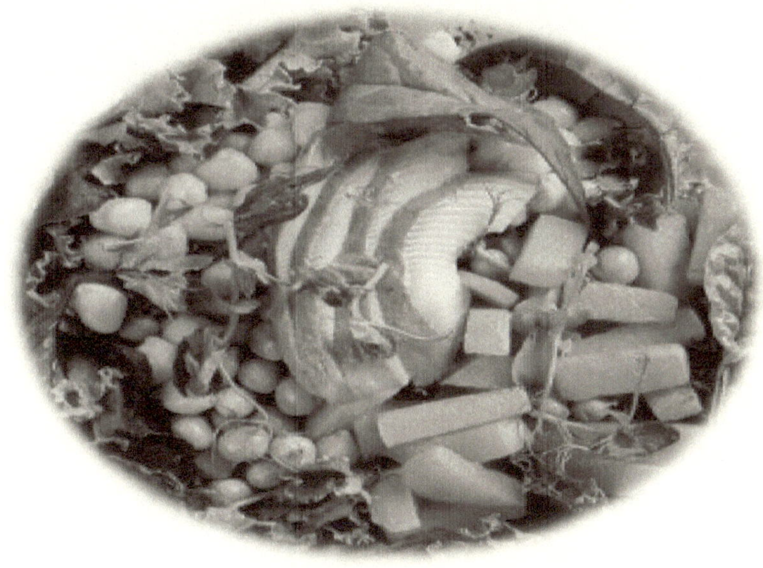

Avocado Papaya Arugula Salad

Prep time: 10 mins
Cook time: 10 mins
Serving: 4
Ingredients:
1 cup of coarsely chopped Arugula
2 (1 cup) of small diced avocado
1/3 cup of chopped unsalted raw Cashew nuts
1/4 cup of coriander Cilantro chopped coarsely or fresh mint
3 tablespoon of fresh Lime juice
4 medium ripe Papaya, divided
2 chopped small shallot
1 finely chopped medium Yellow onion
Preparations:
1. Slice 2 papayas and remove the seeds. Set aside.
2. Peel the other 2 papayas using a vegetable peeler, slice into two and remove the seeds. Dice the peeled and seeded papaya into half-inch sizes, set aside in a bowl.
3. Add shallots, lime juice, cilantro, cashews, and avocados to the peeled and diced papayas, toss together to combine. Season with pepper and salt. Carefully mix in arugula. Serve salad in the papaya halves.

Mixed Vegetables With Pumpkin Dressing

Prep time: 10 mins
Cook time: 13 mins
Servings: 2-3
Ingredients:
2/3 cup of diced carrots
1/2 cup of diced celery
2 middle sized cubed tomatoes
1½ cups of yeast-free vegetable stock
1/2 cup of diced potatoes,
3 tablespoon of lemon juice
2/3 cup of diced broccoli
2/3 cup of diced zucchini
1 sliced spring onion
For the pumpkin dressing:
1/2 cup of pumpkin, cooked
2/3 cup of yeast-free vegetable stock,

1 tablespoon of olive oil
2 tablespoon of lemon juice
1 teaspoon of Dijon-Mustard
Sea salt & pepper
Preparations:
1. Boil the vegetable stock in a medium skillet, and cook potato, celery and carrots, about 8 minutes until soft and firm to the bite. Reserve the stock to cool and set aside.
2. Mix lemon juice with the cooked veggies.
3. Pour zucchini and broccoli into a sieve and steam for about 5 minutes over hot water
4. In a large bowl, combine spring onion, tomato and all other veggies, mix with half or less of the stock.
5. Blend the remaining stock, pumpkin, mustard, oil, lemon juice and salt and pepper.
6. Toss the salad and dressing in a bowl. Serve and enjoy

Vanilla Quinoa Porridge

Prep time: 10 mins
Cook time: 20 mins
Serving: 2
Ingredients:
1/2 teaspoon of fresh grated ground nutmeg
Sprinkle (1/2 a handful) of assorted nuts and seeds of your choice
1-2 drops of vanilla essence
1/2 lemon of skin grated
1/2 cup of coconut cream
1 inch piece of finely grated fresh root ginger or 1 1/2 teaspoons ground ginger
1 stick or 1/2 teaspoon of cinnamon
2 cups of alkaline water
1 cup of dry quinoa, I use organic
Optional: Berries and coconut cream
Preparations:
1. Cook quinoa according to packet instructions. Drain.
2. Pour into the saucepan and stir in the nutmeg, ginger, cinnamon, coconut cream and vanilla essence. Cook for few minutes.

3. Transfer into a big bowl. Serve topped with grated lemon rind and sprinkle with ground cinnamon. Garnish with seeds and nuts of your choice, you can also dollop with coconut cream.

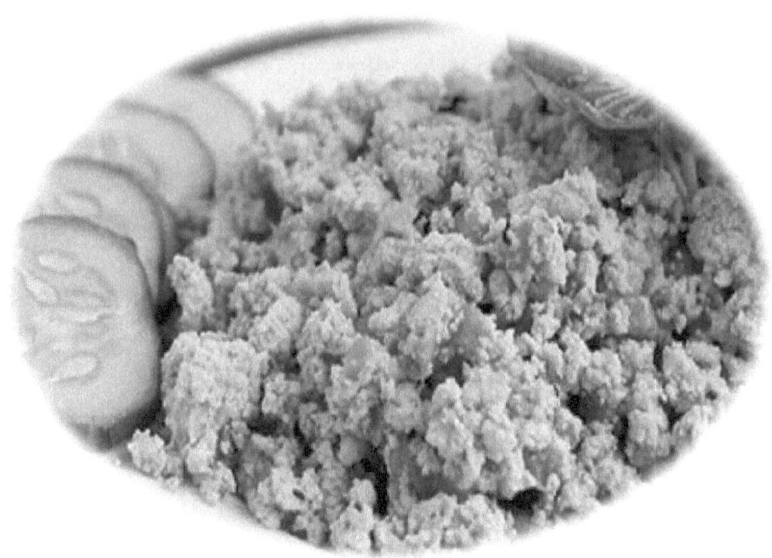

Spiced-up Sprouted Stir-Fry

Prep time: 10 mins

Cook time: 25-30 mins

Serving: 4

Ingredients:

3 cups of filtered water or yeast-free vegetable stock

1 minced garlic clove

1 ½ cup of quinoa, washed and drained

 SAUCE

1 teaspoon of minced ginger

1 minced clove garlic

½ cup of Tamari gluten-free

STIR-FRY

1 handful of mung bean sprouts

½ bunch of kale, cut into ribbons

8 Brussels sprouts, halved

1 stalk celery, cut into chunks

Small head of broccoli, cut into bite size pieces

1 small white onion

2 teaspoons of minced ginger

2 cloves garlic, minced

2 tablespoons of coconut oil

Preparations:

1. Add garlic, vegetable broth and quinoa in a pot and cook the quinoa over high heat.

2. Cover and reduce heat to low when the water comes to a boil, cook for 15-20 minutes or until quinoa is cooked and water is absorbed. Set aside.

For Sauce:

3. Combine the teriyaki ingredients in a small saucepan and simmer until thick and syrupy. Cooking too long will make the sauce salty, so be careful. Set aside

For Stir-Fry:

4. Heat coconut oil in a large pan, add onions, ginger and garlic until brown. Add extra oil if necessary.

5. Add in the vegetables with the exception of sprouts. Stir and cover, cooking for 5 to 10 minutes depending on your desired veggies "al dente".

6. Spoon the quinoa into a bowl; add the stir-fry vegetables in a good amount, then pour in a tablespoon of teriyaki sauce. Top with sprouts. Enjoy!

Vegetables Roast

Prep time: mins

Cook time: mins

Serving: 4

Ingredients:

1/4 cup of pumpkin seeds

Sea salt (Himalayan, Celtic Grey, or Redmond Real Salt)

2 tablespoon of coconut oil

1-2 pounds of the following root vegetables: sweet potatoes, radishes, parsnips, carrots, beets, Turnips, Chopped into bite-sized pieces

Preparations:

1. Toss the vegetables with sea salt and coconut oil, roast for 30 to 40 minutes at 425° F, until slightly browned in spots and soft.

2. Mix sea salt and coconut oil with the pumpkin seeds, and roast together with the vegetables towards the final cooking minutes. Enjoy!

Avocado-Adzuki Bean Stuffed Lettuce Cups

Prep time: mins

Cook time: mins

Serving: 4

Ingredients:

Sea salt (Himalayan, Celtic Grey, or Redmond Real Salt)

1 lime juice

1 avocado

8 butter lettuce leaves or romaine, these make lovely cups

Small handful of chopped cilantro

¼ cup of red onion, minced

1 15-oz can of Adzuki beans, drained and rinsed

Red pepper flakes (optional)

Preparations:

1. In a bowl, mash together the red onion and beans. Add chopped cilantro, stir to combine.

2. Spoon the mash beans into lettuce cups and add diced avocado to the top and with lime juice. Season with red pepper flakes and salt.

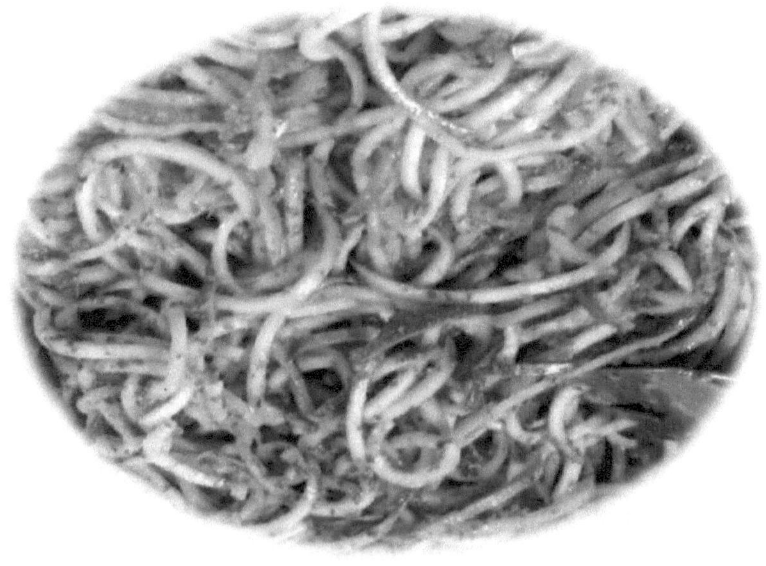

Easy Alkaline Risotto

Prep time: 15 mins
Cook time: 35 mins
Serving: 4

Ingredients:

1 handful of parsley, chopped
1 can of garbanzo beans, rinse thoroughly
2 tablespoons of capers
1 jar artichoke hearts, drained
1 bunch of Swiss chard, cut into ribbons
3 minced cloves garlic
Artichokes medium
1 thinly sliced shallot
2 tablespoon of coconut oil
1 cup of quinoa, rinse and drained
2 cups of yeast free vegetable broth
Salt and pepper (Himalayan, Celtic Grey, or Redmond Real Salt)

Preparations:

1. Add vegetable broth and quinoa in a pot and cook the quinoa over high heat.
2. Cover and reduce heat to low when the water comes to a boil, cook for 20 minutes or until quinoa is cooked and water is absorbed. Set aside.
3. Meanwhile, heat the coconut oil in a sauté pan, add shallots and cook, about 8 minutes until melted. Add Swiss chard and garlic, cook for 5 minutes more. Add artichokes, capers and garbanzo beans and cook for 2 minutes extra.4. Toss the Swiss chard mixture and quinoa in a bowl. Add parsley garnish and season with pepper and sea salt.

Alkaline Cauliflower Rice With Vegetable Curry (Anti-Cancer)

Prep time: 10 mins

Cook time: 10 mins

Servings: 2

Ingredients:

1tbsp of honey

1/2 tsp of cinnamon

1/2 tsp of black pepper

1/2 tsp of turmeric

1/2 tsp of cumin=

1 vegetable stock cube

100g peas - fresh or frozen

2 cabbage leaves, chopped

1 leek, chopped

1 coquette, grated

2 medium tomatoes, slice

200g mushrooms, chop

2 cauliflowers cut into floret chunks

Preparations:

1. Add cauliflower floret into a blender or food processor and blend on low until broken into size of a rice. Set aside in a bowl.

2. For the vegetable curry:

Add the, leek, tomatoes, and mushrooms into a boiling water in a saucepan and simmer for 5 minutes. Drain

3. Combine other vegetables and the drained vegetables into saucepan. Add the stock cube and spices. Stir and simmer for 2 minutes extra. Serve warm.

Haricots Verts With Herbs And Shallots

Prep time: 15 mins

Cook time: 15 mins

Servings: 4

Ingredients:

1/8 tsp of freshly ground black pepper, or more

 1/2 tsp of Celtic sea salt, or more

1/4 cup fresh flat-leaf parsley, loosely packed, chopped coarsely

1/4 cup of fresh mint, loosely packed, chopped coarsely

1/4 cup of lightly toasted sliced almonds

1 lemon finely grated zest and juice

1 1/2 tbsp of unsalted vegan butter

1 lbs. of whole haricots verts

4 small peeled shallots, quartered vertically

1 1/2 tsp of grape seed oil

Preparations:

1. Place a broad cast-iron pot over high-medium heat, then grease with grape seed oil. Lower the heat in case it brings out smokes.

2. Place the cut-side of the shallots down in the pot and let sear, about 4 to 5 minutes until both sides are browned. Set aside in a plate.

3. Working in batches, Cook the beans in batches in the pot, about 8 minutes, tossing not too often, until lightly charred in spots and crisp-tender. Set aside and keep warn while cooking the next batch.

4. Add 1/2 tablespoon of the butter at a time to the beans, along with 1/2 of lemon juice. Toss to coat.

5. Add the shallots and 1/2 parsley, 1/2 almonds, 1/2 mint, and 1/2 lemon zest. Toss to coat, and add salt and pepper to season.

6. Arrange the beans into a serving dish. Sprinkle with the remaining half ingredients. Adjust taste with salt and pepper, Serve warm.

Special Season Broccoli Brussels Sprouts

Prep time: 15 mins

Cook time: 25 mins

Serving: 4

Ingredients:

Fresh cilantro for garnish

2 bunches of greens, as you desire, cut (greens, turnip, escarole, bok choy, collards, kale, etc.)

1 diced onion

4 cups vegetable broth

1 cup of green beans

1 15 ounce can of unsweetened coconut milk

½ cup of snow peas

2 cups of cooked garbanzo beans, or canned

Handful of Brussels sprouts, halved

1 medium crown broccoli, cut into florets

2 tablespoons of green curry paste or powder

Salt to taste

Pepper to taste

2 tablespoons of coconut oil

Preparations:

1. Heat coconut oil in a large pot, add onions and curry spices, sauté about 6-8 minutes or until the onions are soft. Add the beans, coconut milk and vegetables.

2. Simmer on low heat, then add vegetable broth; simmer about 15 minutes until the vegetables are soft. Add in the greens, then add pepper and salt to season. Serve aside quinoa or brown rice. Garnish with cilantro

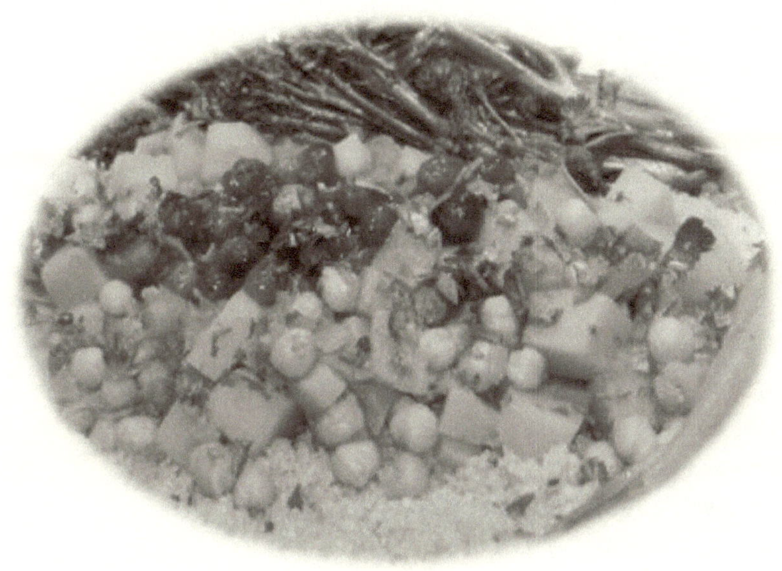

Spaghetti Squash Quinoa Stuffed

Prep time: 60 mins

Cook time: 55 mins

Serves: 2

Ingredients:

1 teaspoon of garlic powder

2 teaspoon of dried thyme

1 1/2 cup of cooked quinoa

Black pepper to taste

1/4 cup of chopped walnuts

2 sliced spring onions, white part

1 red bell pepper, finely chopped

1 medium finely chopped shallot

1 cup of steamed green peas

2 tablespoon of coconut oil

1 big spaghetti squashes, wash and slice in half and seeded

Pink salt to taste

Preparations:

1. Heat up the oven to 400ºF

2. Bake spaghetti squashes, about 40 minutes until tender.

3. Meanwhile heat 1 tablespoon of coconut oil in a skillet and cook the bell pepper and shallot until soft. Add green peas and spices, walnuts and quinoa until heated through. Season with pepper and pink salt.

3. Fill the squash with quinoa walnuts mixture and heat in the oven for 5 – 8 minutes. Serve with fresh greens.

Roasted Cauliflower And Coriander, Turmeric with Mint

Prep time: 15 mins

Cook time: 15 mins

Serving: 4

Ingredients:

1 tablespoon chopped roughly mint

2 tablespoons of chopped roughly coriander/cilantro

1/4 cup of pine nuts

1 large cauliflower, cut into bite size florets

2 teaspoons of ground turmeric (I use organic)

1 tablespoon of ground cumin

Himalayan salt to taste

1/2 cup of coconut oil

Preparations:

1. Heat up the oven to 425F

2. Combine the turmeric, coconut oil, 1/2 teaspoon of salt and cumin in a large bowl, and mix using your hands combine and warm the oil.

3. Add in the cauliflower florets, mix well to coat.

4. Pour the cauliflower on a baking tray, then spread out.

5. Transfer to the pre-warmed oven and roast until the cauliflower is tender and starting to brown, around 15-20 minutes.

6. Meanwhile chuck the pine nuts and slightly toast it on a baking tray in the oven, about a minute.

7. Serve cauliflower in a large bowl and sprinkle with the mint, coriander/cilantro and pine nuts.

Broccoli with Cashew Cream Salad

Prep time: 12

Ready time: S1 hour

Serving: 4

Ingredients:

2 slice of chopped Turkey bacon, cooked

2 tablespoon of hulled   Sunflower seeds

1/4 cup of roughly chopped Cranberries, dried

1/2 cup of roughly chopped Cilantro (coriander)

1/4 cup of diced Red onion

3/4 tablespoon of roughly chopped Cashew nuts, roasted

4 cup of Broccoli, cut into small sizes

For Dressing

4 teaspoon of Curry powder

5 1/2 teaspoon of Water

1/2 teaspoon of Salt

3/4 cup of Cashew nuts, roasted, salted

2 1/2 teaspoon of Agave nectar (syrup)

1 tablespoon of Apple cider vinegar

1 dash   Black pepper

Preparations:

1. Cover the cashews in a bowl of water and refrigerate for 8 hours. Drain.

2. Place the drained cashew into a small food processor, add the dressing ingredients and blend until smooth and creamy. Set aside.

3. Combine the turkey bacon, cranberries, red onion, broccoli and cilantro in a large bowl. Stir well to combine. Cover and allow sitting for not less than an hour. Mix in the cashews and sunflower seeds, just before serving. Enjoy!

Prep time: 10 mins

Cook time: 0 mins

Serving: 4

Ingredients:

1 tablespoon of Nutritional yeast

1/4 cup of Lemon juice

3 cup of chopped Kale

1/2 cup of hulled Hemp seeds, shelled

2 minced Garlic cloves

1/4 cup of olive oil, extra virgin

1/2 cup of canned Artichoke hearts

1/8 teaspoon of Salt and pepper

Preparations:

1. Add the ingredients in a food processor, adding the garlic lastly. Season with the pepper and salt. Pulse until your desired consistency is reached.

2. Serve the pesto over pasta or zucchini noodles, a dip for crackers, on toast or veggies.

Store unused portions in the refrigerator in a glass airtight container for a week.

SNACKS RECIPES

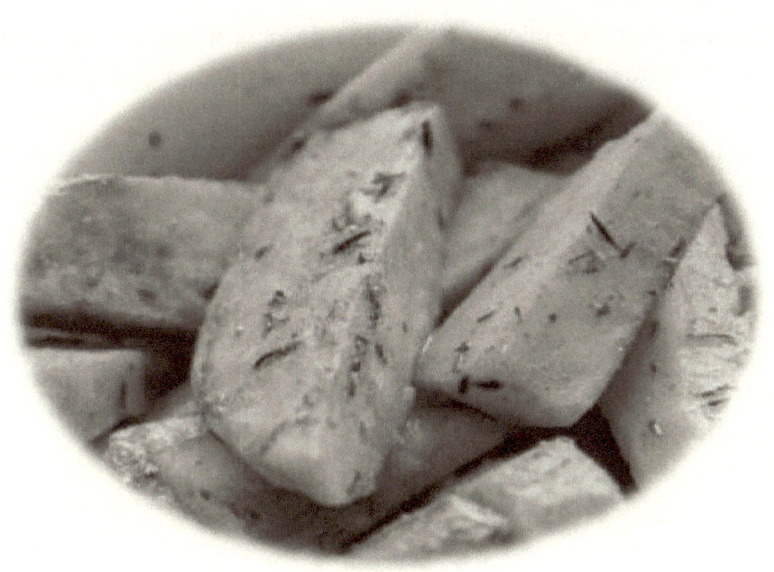

Cucumber Bites with Tuna Mix

Prep time: 15 mins

Cook time: 0 mins

Serving: 12

Ingredients:

1 can of white tuna, canned in water, drained

1 whole fresh lime juice (divided)

1 minced Garlic clove

2 teaspoon of extra virgin olive oil

1 (12 sliced) Cucumber

3 tomato Cherry Tomatoes (for garnish)

3 tomato diced Cherry Tomatoes

1 pinch of Salt and pepper

1 peeled, pitted Avocado

Preparations:

1. Mix the olive oil, drained tuna, and half lime juice together in a small bowl. Season with pepper and salt. Set aside.

2. Mash the remaining lime juice and avocado flesh with fork until partially smooth in a different small bowl. Mix in diced tomatoes and minced garlic. Season with salt and pepper.

3. Lay out cucumber slices on. Spoon small tuna mixture on each cucumber slice and cherry tomato quarter on a serving tray. Enjoy!

Apple Collard Coconut vinegar Wrap

Ready time: 5

Servings: 4

Ingredients:

1 cup of Walnuts or pecans

1 thinly sliced sweet onion

1/8 teaspoon of Sea salt (to taste)

4 leaf of Collard greens

1/8 teaspoon of Coconut vinegar (to taste)

2 thinly sliced medium Apple

Preparations:

1. Slice the leaves into two and discard the hard stem.

2. Stuff each half green with ingredients, wrap and enjoy!

Alkaline Tasty Raw Chili

Serving: 2

Ingredients:

½ teaspoon of sea salt

1 teaspoon of cumin

1 tablespoons of chili powder

¼ chopped yellow onion

¼ yellow squash

½ red bell pepper

2 tablespoons of olive oil

2 tablespoons of finely chopped garlic

6 sun-dried tomatoes

1 large tomato

Preparations:

1. Transfer every ingredient into a food processor with "S" blade, pulse some couple of times to chop ingredients, then blend until your desired consistency is reached.

2. You can allow sit for an hour to let all of the spices mesh together before serving or serve immediately.

California Chia Pudding

Prep time: 15 mins

Serving: 4

Ingredients:

2 tablespoons of Chia seeds, ground

1 cup of Almond milk, vanilla, unsweetened, Silk

1 cup of cubes   Papaya

1 large Banana

3 tablespoon of Coconut, shredded, unsweetened

1 tsp of Cinnamon

Preparations:

1. Pour almond milk in a bowl, add chia seeds to soak for about 10 minutes.

2. Mix the remaining ingredients, reserving 1 tablespoon of coconut with the chia mixture in a food processor or blender, blend until smooth.

3. Serve right away into 4 individual bowl and add the remaining shredded coconut to the top or chill in the refrigerator before serving.

Alkaline Tasty Jalapenos Poppers

Prep time: 15 mins

Cook time: 5 hours

Serving: 16 Jalapenos

Ingredients:

16 Jalapenos

½ garlic clove

6 medium pitted dates

1 tsp of Celtic sea salt

2 tbs of apple cider vinegar

1 tbs of lemon juice

1 large avocado

1 cup of pine nuts

Preparations:

1. Combine the dates, pine nuts and garlic in a food processor, blend until smooth. Then add avocado flesh, lemon juice and sea salt, blend lightly.

2. Slit the jalapenos from the side or cut from the top, scoop out the seeds.

3. Stuff the jalapenos with the mix.

4. Transfer the stuffed jalapenos on a baking pan place in the oven, about 5 hours at 105 F or until tender.

Tuna And Kale Stuffed Avocado

Prep time: 15 mins

Cook time: 10 mins

Serving: 2

Ingredients:

1 Avocado, pitted and halved

1 teaspoon of Soy sauce

1 teaspoon of extra virgin olive oil

1 tablespoon of chopped scallion, Green onion,

114 grams of White tuna, canned in water, drained

1 cup of finely chopped Kale

Preparations:

1. Pour olive oil into a sauté pan and sauté the scallions for 3 to 4 minutes. Stir in tuna, and sauté for 2 more minutes.

2. Add in the soy sauce and kale. Cover and cook for 3 to 4 minutes.

3. Fill each avocado half with the mixture.

Alkaline Mashed Avocado Wraps

Prep time: 5 mins

Servings: 2

Ingredients:

1 organic lemon juice

1/2 bunch of chopped fresh coriander or parsley

½ fresh chopped chilli

½ medium-sized chopped red onion

3 ripe avocados

2 ripe chopped tomatoes

6 big romaine lettuce leaves,

1 pinch Himalayan crystal salt

Preparations:

1. Mash the avocados in a bowl using a fork until fine.

2. Add lemon juice and salt over the mashed avocado and mix in the parsley, coriander red onion, and tomatoes.

3. Wash the lettuce leaves and them pat dry.

4. Scoop the mixture over the lettuce leaves, wrap and keep intact with a cocktail stick!

Alkaline Pumpkin Fries

Prep time: 10 mins

Cook time: 30-40 mins

Servings: 1 tray

Ingredients:

Pinch of cumin powder

½ teaspoon of cayenne pepper

1 teaspoon of organic or sea salt

¼ cup of extra virgin olive oil (cold pressed)

Pinch of curry powder

1 pumpkin

Preparations:

1. Heat up the oven to 350° F.

2. Slice pumpkin into two, discard seeds and strings, wash well and peel out the large pieces with a sharp knife. Slice the pulp just like a French Fries.

3. Lay the pumpkin slices on a tray, carefully pour in olive oil or spray with an oil sprayer, and then season with cumin powder, curry powder, pepper and salt.
4. Place in the preheated oven and bake for 30 to 40 minutes, toss occasionally.

Gallant Grilled Veggies

Prep time: 10 mins
Cook time: 20-30 mins
Servings: 4
Ingredients:
Fresh herbs, (like basil, thyme, oregano) chopped
3 tbsp. cold pressed extra virgin olive oil
2 crushed garlic cloves
1 big diced onion
4 diced carrots
1 green bell pepper
1 yellow bell pepper
1 diced red bell pepper, into bite-sized pieces
1 big diced eggplants, into bite-sized pieces
1 big diced zucchini, into bite-sized pieces
Sea salt and freshly ground pepper
Preparations:
1. Preheat oven to 350°F.
2. Combine the veggies in a large bowl, mix in the olive oil to coat the veggies are lightly.
3. Transfer the veggies to a baking sheet. Add salt and pepper to season then drizzle with herbs.
4. Place in the oven and grill for 20-30 minutes at 325°F.

Prep time: 5 mins

Servings: 2

Ingredients:

2 tablespoon of water cress

2 tablespoon of chives, fresh

½ lemon, juiced

1 peel and diced celery root

1 diced spring onion

1 diced carrot

2 peel kohlrabis, cut in thinly slices

3 tablespoon of extra virgin olive oil

Salt & pepper

Preparations:

1. Combine onions, carrot, and celery in a salad bowl and stir well.

2. Combine cress, chives, pepper, salt and lemon juice, and mix with vegetables.

3. Arrange kohlrabis slices on two plates and pour the vegetable mixture over kohlrabi slices.

Alkalizing Green Pasta

Prep time: 20 mins

Cook time: 20 mins

Serving: 2

Ingredients:

1 medium leek (sliced into thinly rounds, rinsed)

1 cup of raw or frozen Green peas

1 minced Garlic cloves

1/2 tablespoon of olive oil or Coconut oil

3 peeled, julienned large Carrots, into spaghetti-like strands

1 bunch of Asparagus, trimmed and chopped into one-inch pieces

For Pesto

1 tablespoon of Water

1/4 cup of Sun-dried tomato, packed in oil, drained

1/4 teaspoon of Sea salt

1 tablespoon of Lemon juice

1 Garlic clove

3/4 cup of fresh Basil

2 tablespoon of extra virgin olive oil

1/4 cup of hulled Hemp seeds, shelled

Preparations:

1. Cover the julienned carrots with a damp paper towel so it won't dry out.

2. Heat up oil in a large pan over medium. Sauté the garlic and sliced leek for 3-4 minutes, until tender. Add salt and plenty grounds of pepper.

3. Add asparagus and sauté, until tender, about 8 minutes more. Mix in the peas and cook for few more minutes until heated through.

4. Mince the garlic in a food processor, add in the sun-dried tomatoes and basil and blend until smooth.

5. Add the remaining pesto ingredients and process until finely combined.

6. Mix the pesto into the pan containing vegetable mixture, cook until heated through. Add Seasoning to taste. To serve, pour the vegetable pesto mix over the carrot pasta.

Winter Indoor Timely Pasta

Prep time: 10 mins

Cook time: 35 mins

Serving: 4

Ingredients:

1 can of garbanzo beans, rinsed and drained (optional)

1 sprig of rosemary, chopped

1 handful of parsley, chopped

1 thinly sliced leek

½ tsp of red pepper flakes (optional)

1 package of kelp noodles

3 minced garlic cloves

3 tablespoons of olive oil, extra virgin or coconut oil

1 medium of broccoli head

Salt and pepper

Preparations:

1. Warm up the oven to 400 F. Combine broccoli, red pepper flakes, olive oil, salt, and garlic in a bowl, toss to coat. Roast in the oven for 20 minutes until soft.

2. Rinse kelp noodles and also drain it, then soak in a pot of hot water.

3. Meanwhile, in a sauté pan, heat 2 tablespoons of oil, and cook leeks, about 8 minutes until melted.

4. Drain and add the kelp noodles to the leeks. Cooking for about 7 to 8 minutes. Add broccoli, rosemary, parsley, pepper and salt.

Add garbanzo beans if using.

Perfect Marinated Zucchini Squash

Prep time: 10 mins
Cook time: 60 mins
Serving: 4
Ingredients:
1 tablespoon of minced basil
1 tablespoon of minced dill
1 tablespoon of minced oregano
1 tablespoon of olive oil
½ cup of sun-dried tomatoes, chopped
2 fresh yellow squash
2 fresh zucchini, slice and squash thin into half mooned shape sizes
1 teaspoon of sea salt
Preparations:
1. Place the zucchini in a bowl and add the remaining ingredients, toss and allow
the vegetables marinate for 30 minutes to 1 hour or steam or sauté for 4 minutes
or grill for few minute

SOUP RECIPES

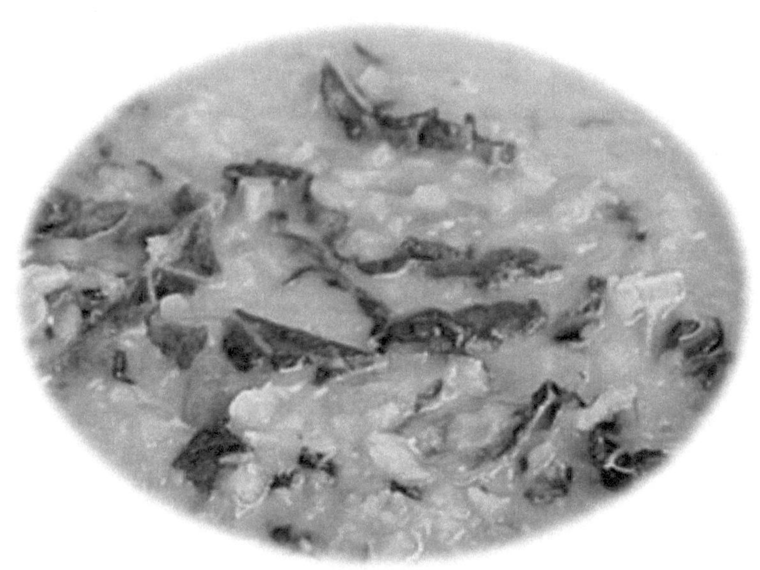

Creamy Citrus- Cilantro Dressing

Prep time: 5 mins

Servings: 1

Ingredients:

1 tsp of agave juice

½ cup of olive oil

1 tbs of cayenne powder

1 tbs of shallots, chopped

2 tbs of green onion, chopped

2 tbs of cilantro, chopped

1 tbs of lime juice

1 cup of orange juice

½ avocado

Preparations:

1. Combine all the ingredients in a food processor reserving the olive oil. Blend until smooth. Add the olive oil and blend more for 30 seconds.

2. Serve with your favorite salad.

Spinach Broccoli And Ginger Soup

Prep time: 10 mins

Cook time: 25 mins

Serving: 4

Ingredients:

1/4 tsp of Black pepper

4 cup of chopped Broccoli

2 medium chopped Celery stalk

1 tablespoon of extra virgin olive oil

2 chopped Garlic cloves

1 tablespoon of minced Ginger root

2 teaspoon of Lemon juice to taste

1/2 cup of roughly chopped fresh Parsley

3 parsnips peeled, cored, chopped

1/4 teaspoon of Sea salt to taste

7 cup of Spinach

4 cup of Water

Preparations:

1. Heat olive oil in a large pot over medium heat and stir in the onion, ginger and garlic. Add the parsley, celery, parsnips, spinach and broccoli and stir briefly until the spinach is wilted.

2. Add the necessary measure of water needed to cover the vegetables at first. You can add more water to thin the soup out later.

3. Simmer on high, cover and simmer on medium heat, about 15 minutes or until the veggies are tender.

4. Puree the soup with an immersion blender add a squeeze of citrus.

Kale Soup With Creamy Red Lentil

Prep time: 5 mins

Cook time: 50 mins

Serving: 6

Ingredients:

1/2 medium diced Yellow onion

2 3/4 cup of Vegetable stock

2 tablespoons of canned tomato sauce

1 teaspoon of Sea salt

3 diced Roma tomatoes Kale

1 1/2 cup of Red lentils, raw

1 cup of chopped Kale

1 1/2 teaspoon of Cumin

1 (13.5 oz) can of Coconut milk

1/4 teaspoon of Cayenne pepper

Preparations:

1. Combine all ingredients, reserving the coconut milk and chopped kale into a medium pot, stir and cook until heated through.

2. Reduce heat to medium-low and simmer with the lid on, stirring occasionally for 30 - 40 minutes or until the lentils are tender.

3. Turn heat off heat, add coconut milk and chopped kale, stir well.

Adjust salt, if needed. Enjoy!

Chilled Avocado, Watercress Soup

Prep time: 5 mins

Cook time: 2 mins

Serving: 1

Ingredients:

Cherry tomatoes, halved to garnish

Pepper to taste

2 scallions

1 ½ cups of filtered water

2 freshly squeezed lemons

2 cups of watercress

Salt to taste

1 cup of diced cucumber

3 organic Haas avocados

Preparations:

1. Combine all ingredients in a bowl to a puree. Add some pepper and salt to taste, then garnish with the cherry tomatoes.

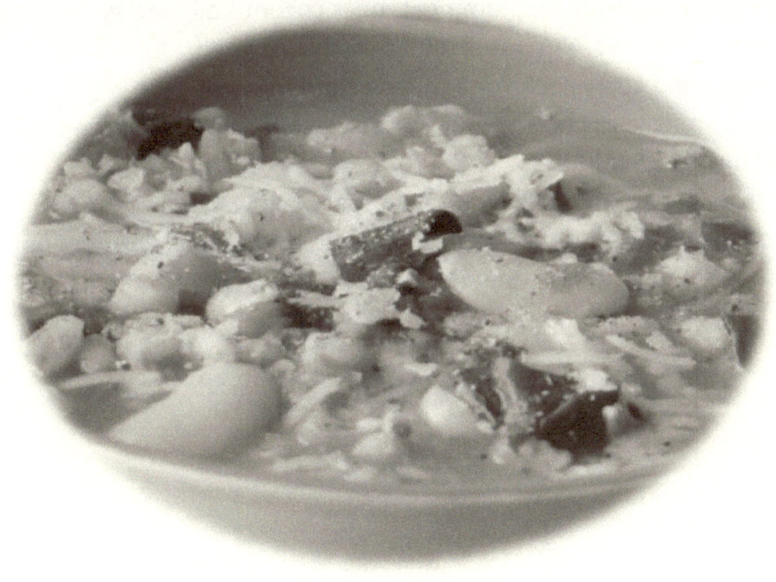

Curry Powder Carrot Soup

Prep time: mins

Cook time: mins

Serving: 4

Ingredients:

1/2 bunch of chopped cilantro

2 cups of filtered water

1 15oz can of full-fat coconut milk

3 cups of carrots cut into 1-inch sizes

1 teaspoon of turmeric

2 teaspoons of curry powder

1 lime juice and zest

4 minced cloves garlic

1 1/2 inch piece of ginger, sliced and crushed

1 tablespoon of coconut oil

Sea salt and black pepper to taste

Preparations:

1. In a large saucepan over medium heat, heat coconut oil, Add garlic, lime zest and ginger and cook, about 3-4 minutes until slightly browned.

2. Add turmeric and curry cook for a minute until fragrant.

3. Add coconut milk, carrots, and water. Cook to heat through, then simmer low with the lid on, for 15 minutes.

4 Remove from heat and let sit for 30 minutes to allow flavors to meld.

5. Puree soup using a food processor or blender, and season with pepper and salt. Garnish with lime juice and chopped cilantro, Enjoy!

Healthy Healing Soup

Prep time: 15 mins

Cook time: 25 mins

Serving: 4

Ingredients:

1 tablespoon of coconut oil

200ml, magnesium-free, yeast-free vegetable stock

1 brown onion, roughly chopped

4 garlic cloves, roughly chopped

1 handful of roughly chopped cashews

2 tablespoon of chopped dill

1 red bell pepper, roughly chopped and deseeded

2 carrots, chopped

1 large handful of spinach

1 large sweet potato, chopped

1 avocado

1 can (200g) lentils (drained and washed)

Preparations:

1. Heat coconut oil in a large saucepan, and sauté the garlic and onion.
 Add carrots, and sweet potato into the pan, stir to combine, about 2 minutes.
2. Add in vegetable stock, and simmer until the vegetables are just soft but not overcooked, about 10 minutes. Add the lentils, simmer for 5 minutes.
3. If you don't have a big blender, you will have to do this in batches. Transfer into a blender and add in the dill, spinach, capsicum, and avocado. Reserve a few sprigs of dill back for garnish.
4. Puree until smooth. Serve with sprigs of dill, sprinkle with the cashews.

Broccoli-Creamy Avocado Soup

Prep time: 10 mins

Cook time: 15 mins

Servings: 4

Ingredients:

Some fresh cilantro, basil, cumin to taste

Celtic Sea Salt to taste

2 cups of yeast-free vegetable broth

1 celery stalk

1 green or red pepper

1 chopped yellow onion

1 small avocado

2-3 chopped broccoli flowers

Preparations:

1. Warm up the vegetable broth (do not cook).

2. Add chopped broccoli and onion, and heat until broccoli is soft.

3. Transfer into the blender, add the celery, pepper and avocado, and puree until you have a creamy soup is creamy (add water if too thick).

Fresh Harvest Vegetable Soup

Prep time: 10 mins

Cook time: 10 mins

Servings: 4

Ingredients:

Alkaline Carrot Soup

1 tablespoon of fresh basil

4-5 tablespoon of yeast-free vegetable broth

1 quart of (alkaline) water

1 yellow onion

3 stalks of chopped asparagus

1 cup of chopped broccoli

1 celery stalk

1 small chopped zucchini

2 large carrots

2 tablespoon of sea salt to taste

Preparations:

1. Pour water into a pot, add onion and vegetable broth, bring to a boil.

2. Shred the celery stalk and carrots in a food processor and set aside with the asparagus, zucchini, and broccoli.

3. Turn heat off once the water is boiling to avoid boiling the vegetables. Add celery stalk, carrots, asparagus, zucchini, and broccoli into the hot water and allow to soften as desired.

4. Let cool slightly, then puree in the blender until you get a smooth and thick consistency. Adjust taste with salt, Enjoy while it's warm.

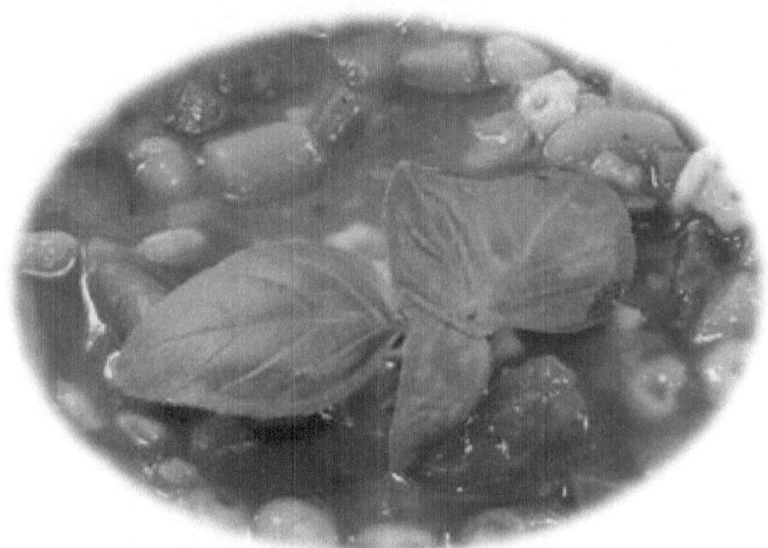

White Bean With Pumpkin And Sage Soup

Prep time: 15 mins

Cook time: 45 mins

Servings: 4

Ingredients:

1 ½ quart water (preferably alkaline water)

1 tablespoon of sage

1 tablespoon of your favorite herbs, slice in fine pieces

1 tablespoon of cold pressed extra virgin olive oil

2 cloves of garlic, slice in fine pieces

1 onion, slice in fine pieces

½ pound of white beans

½ pound of sweet potatoes, cut in cubes

1 ½ pound pumpkin, cut in cubes

A pinch of pepper and sea salt

Preparations:

1. Add olive oil in a sauce pan, Stir-fry the garlic and onion for a couple of minutes.

2. Add the sage, herbs, pumpkin and potatoes and fry for another 5 minutes.
3. Add water and cook with the lid on, about 30 minutes or until vegetables are soft.
4. Add beans, pepper and salt. Cook for 5 more minutes. Serve and enjoy!

Cauliflower-Swiss Emmenthal-Soup

Prep time: 10 mins
Cook time: 10 mins
Servings: 2

Ingredients:

2 cups of cauliflower pieces
1 cup of potatoes, cut in cubes
2 cups of yeast-free vegetables stock
3 tablespoon of Swiss Emmenthal cheese, cut in cubes
2 tablespoon of fresh chives
1 tablespoon of pumpkin seeds
1 pinch of cayenne pepper and nutmeg
Salt and pepper (optional)

Preparations:

1. Warm vegetable stock in a soup pot and cook the potato and cauliflower for 5-6 minutes or until soft, and then puree with a blender.
2. Season with and cayenne pepper and nutmeg, and salt and pepper (optional).
3. Add fresh chives and emmenthal cheese and stir for some minutes until the soup is smooth. Garnish with pumpkin seeds.

Greek Lentils Flaky Soup

Prep time: 10 mins

Cook time: 1 hour 10 mins

Servings: 4

Ingredients:

½ teaspoon of oregano

1 bay leaf

1 tablespoon of fresh lime or lemon juice

2 tablespoon of extra virgin olive oil, cold-pressed

3-4 diced garlic cloves

1 diced onion

½ stalk of leek, cut very fine slices

1 carrot, cut very fine slices

2 big tomatoes, Puree

½ pound small lentils

Pinch of sea salt and pepper to taste

Preparations:

1. Rinse the lentils and drain. Then add into a bowl of water to soak overnight. Rinse lentils and drain again in the next day.

2. Bring the lentils to boil for 5 minutes. Drain and set aside.

3. In a big pot, Pour 4 cups of water. Add the bay leave, tomatoes, leek, carrots, garlic and onions and bring to boil.

4. Add lentils, lower heat and simmer covering partially for up to 1 hour. Adjust thickness with water if necessary.

5. Lastly, add the lemon/lime juice and olive oil, then season with oregano, salt, pepper.

Easy Alkaline Porridge

Prep time: 3 mins
Cook time: 4 mins
Serving: 1
Ingredients:
2-3 tablespoons of cranberries or dried cherries
1/4 teaspoon of alcohol free vanilla
Powdered stevia to taste
Cinnamon to taste
1/3 cup thin flaked spelt, preferably
1 cup of filtered water
Toppings:
Raw nuts, seeds, hemp nuts, fresh raspberries, blueberries, blackberries or strawberries
1/2 cup of hazelnut, unsweetened almond, rice milk or hemp
Preparations:
1. Combine the ingredients together in a pot and simmer over medium heat, about 3-4 mins, Transfer into a large bowl.
2. Pour almond or hazelnut or any non-dairy milk. Enjoy!

Cucumber- Avocado Sushi Rolls

Prep time: 15 mins
Cook time: 15 mins
Servings: 1
Ingredients:
1 Cucumber
Guacamole
1/8 tsp of sweet paprika, to garnish
Pinch of cayenne pepper, and more
1/4 tsp of ground cumin, and more
1/4 tsp of Celtic sea salt, and more
1 tbsp of fresh lemon juice, and more
1 cup of curly kale leaves, removed ribs, chiffonaded
1 peeled and pitted large avocado
Preparations:
1. Slice the zucchini using a wide vegetable peeler or 16-inch setting on a mandolin and cut long slices straight down on one side (until you reach the seeds), another

long slices straight down over the second side. Remove the outer green layers. Set aside.

2. Mash the avocado, and stir in the, lemon juice, chopped kale leaves, cayenne, and cumin, salt and in a bowl together. Tweak cayenne, cumin, salt and lemon juice to taste.

3. To assemble: spread on each cucumber strip, quarter of the mixture, and carefully roll up into fine round roll. (Secure with a skewer.)

4. Arrange the rolls onto a plate end down, and sprinkle smoked paprika over it. Consume immediately.

SALADS RECIPES

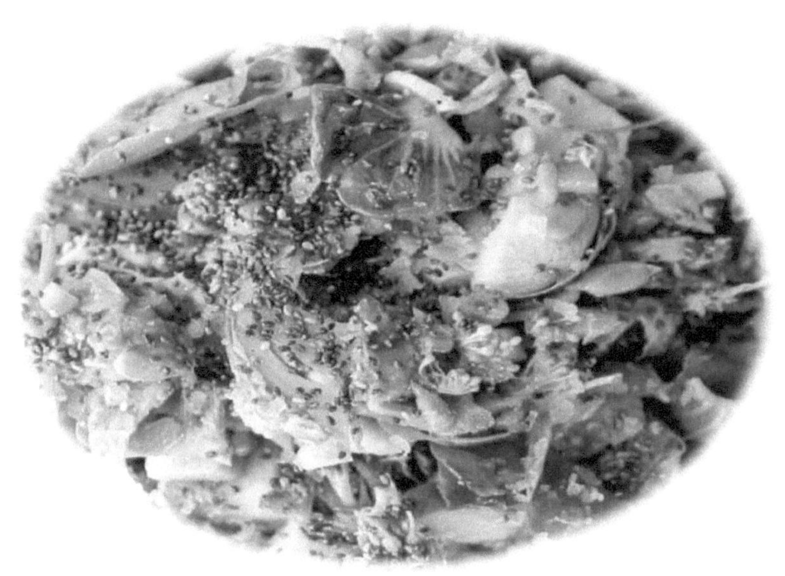

Avocado Cole Slaw Dressing

Prep time: 10 mins

Cook time: 3 mins

Servings: 1

Ingredients:

Cayenne pepper and dash of sea salt to taste

1 fresh lemon, juice

3-4 tablespoon of cold pressed extra virgin olive oil

1 avocado

3 tablespoon of parsley, chopped

1 small red onion, shredded

1 tomato, chopped

2 carrots, shredded

½ cup of red or green cabbage, shredded

Preparations:

1. Combine the carrots and cabbage, and parsley, tomato and onion and the in a big bowl.

2. Blend the fresh lemon juice, olive oil and avocado, and pour over the salad.

3. Add Cayenne pepper and sea salt to taste. Enjoy!

Avocado Apple Sesame Salad

Prep time: 15 mins

Cook time: 15 mins

Servings: 2

Ingredients:

1/2 tsp of sesame seeds, and more

1 tsp of cilantro, finely chopped

1 avocado, cut in half, and pitted

Pinch of red pepper flakes

1/4 tbsp of garlic powder

1/4 tbsp of onion powder

1/4 tbsp of Celtic sea salt, and more to serve

1 1/2 tsp of minced fresh ginger

1 tbsp of toasted sesame oil

2 tbsp of fresh lemon juice

1 finely diced green apple

Preparation:

1. Combine the sesame oil, ginger, lemon juice, apple, red pepper flakes, garlic powder, onion powder and salt in a bowl.

2. Fill each avocado cavity evenly with apple mixture. Garnish with sesame seeds and cilantro. Serve immediately.

Healthy Brussels Sprouts

Prep time: 30 mins

Cook time: 30 mins

Servings: 6-8

Ingredients:

Dressing:

1/8 tsp of red pepper flakes

1/2 tsp of Celtic sea salt or Massel chicken-flavored seasoning powder

2 tsp of minced garlic (2 cloves)

1 1/2 tsp of Dijon mustard

1 1/2 tsp of Bragg liquid aminos

1 1/2 tbsp of sweet white

1/4 cup (40g) raw sunflower seeds, soaked

1/4 cup of raw pine nuts, soaked, (40g)

1/4 cup of fresh lemon juice, (60ml)

1 cup of vegetable broth or Massel chicken-flavored, (240ml)

Salad:

1/4 cup shelled hemp seeds, (35g)

1 cup blanched slivered almonds, (140g) or 1 cup sprouted watermelon seeds, (130g)

5 cups shaved Brussels sprouts, (400g)

5 cups shredded white cabbage, (500g)

Preparations:

1. Combine all ingredients for the dressing into your blender and blend for 30 to 60 seconds on high, until smooth.

2. Stir the cabbage and Brussels sprouts together in a large salad bowl. Pour 1/2 of the mixture and toss until well coated. Stir in more dressing. Toss with hemp seeds and the almonds or watermelon seeds.

3. Serve with the remaining dressing.

Healthy Fresh Vegetable Salad

Prep time: 10 mins

Cook time: 3 mins

Servings: 1

Ingredients:

1 head romaine lettuce

2 chopped tomatoes

2 shredded carrots

1 diced red bell pepper

1 diced green bell pepper

1 diced small cucumber

1 thinly sliced red onion

Alkalizing Citrus Salad Dressing

Preparations:

1. Combine salad ingredients into a bowl and stir together. Pour the dressing over the salad. Enjoy!

Tofu Broccoli Salad

Prep time: 10 mins

Cook time: 25 mins

Servings: 2

Ingredients:

1 tablespoon of fresh lemon juice

2 tablespoon of soy sauce

5 tablespoon of cold pressed olive oil

2 flowers of broccoli

300g organic tofu

Sea salt to taste

Pepper to taste

1 clove garlic

½ red pepper bell

Preparations:

1. Heat olive oil in a pan and fry the diced tofu in it for about 15 minutes. Turn heat off, and then pour the soy sauce over the tofu. Transfer into a bowl.

2. Fry the broccoli, stirring frequently for 10 minutes until soft. Allow to cool.

3. Pour the fresh lime juice, olive oil, pepper, garlic and salt, in a blender and blend until smooth.

4. Transfer broccoli into the tofu bowl, then pour the dressing over, stir.
5. Add red pepper bell slices to garnish. Enjoy!

Carrot-Fennel With Pomegranate Salad

Prep time: 5 mins
Cook time: 5 mins
Servings: 2

Ingredients:

1 fennel bulb, Slice into strips
1 ½ cup grated carrots
1 tablespoon of olive oil extra virgin
5 tablespoons of fresh orange juice
3 tablespoons of fresh lemon juice
1 pomegranate
Fresh pepper
Salt

Preparations:

1. Cut the outside of the pomegranate and get out seeds and flesh.
2. Mix orange juice, 1 ½ tablespoon of lemon juice, and pepper, salt and oil in a salad bowl. Add carrots and pomegranate and stir well.
3. Stir 2 tbsp water, remaining lemon juice, fennel and small amount of salt in a separate bowl.
4. Combine mixture together, and serve on plates.

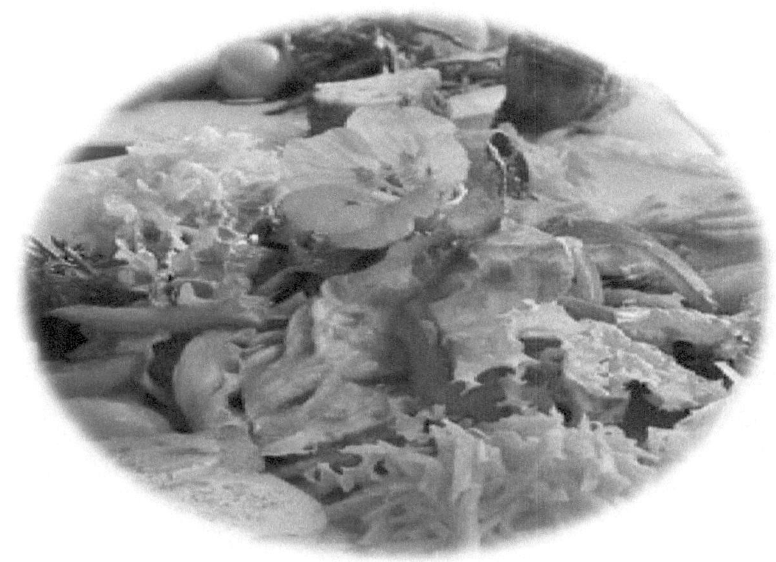

Alkaline Almond Celery- Salad

Prep time: 5 mins

Cook time: 5 mins

Servings: 1 bowl

Ingredients:

1/2 lemon

1/3 cup of almonds

 2/3 cup of water

6-7 ounces of cubed apple

10 ounces of sliced knob celery

Pepper

1/2 TL salt

Preparations:

1. Mix lemon juice, apples and celery in a large bowl.

2. Blend water and almonds until smooth.

3. Pour almond mix, pepper and salt into the bowl, stir well to combine, then store in refrigerator for 1 hour.

Prep time: 5 mins

Cook time: 5 mins

Servings: 2

Ingredients:

Fresh basil leaves

1 small stalk of leek, diced into fine stripes

5-6 black olives, diced into fine stripes

1 red bell pepper, diced

1 cup of cherry tomatoes, halved

2 cups of roman lettuce

Salad dressing:

Pinch of fresh pepper

½ teaspoon of dried basil

½ teaspoon of ground oregano

¼ teaspoon of garlic powder

Pinch of sea salt

2 tablespoon of cold pressed extra virgin olive oil

2 tablespoon of fresh lemon or lime juice

1 tbsp. of flaxseeds, optional for thicker dressing

Preparations:

1. Cut the roman lettuce and basil leaves in pieces of medium sizes. Add olives, peppers, tomatoes, leek, and bell pepper in a big salad bowl.

2. Combine the salad ingredients dressing in a blender and blend until smooth. Adjust the season as desired.

3. Toss the salad and dressing in a bowl. Serve and enjoy

Alkaline Intercontinental Salad

Prep time: 5 mins

Cook time: 5 mins

Servings: 2

Ingredients:

Celery leaves, chopped

1 small stalk of leek, chopped

1 onion, chopped

10 black olives in oil

3 large tomatoes, diced

1 each red and yellow bell pepper, diced

For the salad dressing:

Pinch of cayenne pepper

½ teaspoon of ground cumin

1 teaspoon of dried basil

¼ teaspoon of dried rosemary

½ teaspoon of ground oregano

1 teaspoon of garlic powder

3/4 cup of cold pressed olive oil

Pinch of sea salt

1/3 cup of fresh lemon plus or lime juice

1 tbsp. of flaxseeds, optional for thicker dressing

Preparations:

1. Combine the finely chopped and diced salad ingredients in a salad bowl.
Prepare the salad dressing:

2. Combine the salad ingredients dressing in a blender and blend until smooth.
Adjust the season as desired.

3. Toss the salad and dressing in a bowl. Serve and enjoy

Avocado Wild Garlic Salad

Prep time: 5 mins

Cook time: 5 mins

Servings: 2

Ingredients:

1 avocado, peeled and cut in thin slices

1 bunch of wild garlic, chopped in fine pieces

3 chopped tomatoes

1 red pepper bell, peeled and cut in thin slices

2 tbsp. of extra virgin olive oil, coldpressed

Organic salt to taste

Pinch of cayenne pepper

Preparations:

1. Combine everything in a medium-sized bowl.

2. Pour pepper, salt and olive oil, mix well.

DESSERT

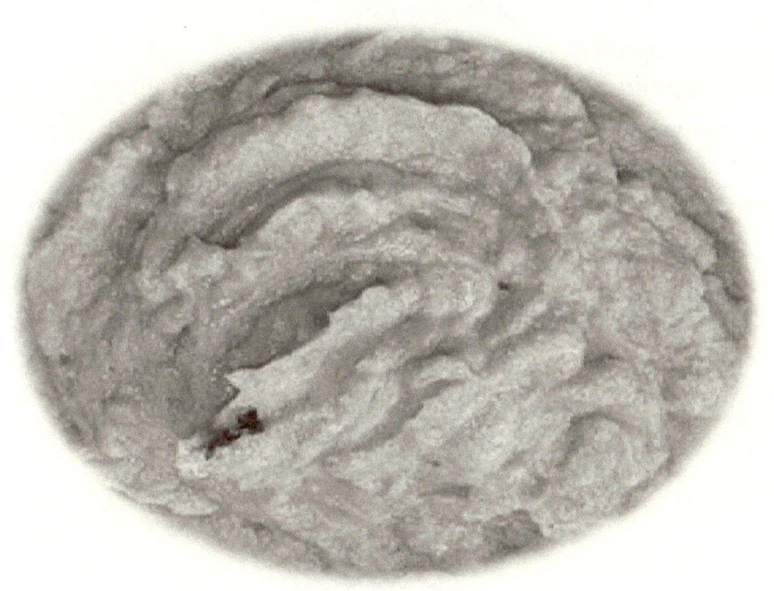

Alkaline Avocado Chocolate

Servings: 2

Ingredients:

1½ teaspoon of Celtic Sea Salt

3-5 dates

2 tablespoons of raw cacao

1 tablespoon of vanilla

2/3 cup of coconut water, preferably raw

1½ of Haas avocado

Preparations:

1. Blend ingredients in blender on high and refrigerate to firm up.

Alkaline Raw Chocolate Pudding

Servings: 4

Ingredients:

Unsweetened shredded coconut for garnish

2-3 tablespoon of coconut milk

1 teaspoon of coconut oil

1 teaspoon of lemon juice

1 tablespoon of raw honey

3 tablespoon of raw cacao powder

2 bananas, chopped and/or 1 chopped avocado

Preparations:

1. Blend all ingredients together with the exception of shredded coconut and coconut milk. Slowly pour in coconut milk until the desired consistency is reached. Sprinkled with shredded coconut. Serve and enjoy!

Alkaline Luxury Figs

Servings: 4

Ingredients:

4 tablespoon of cup raw honey

4 tablespoon of walnuts, toasted and chopped

¼ teaspoon of cinnamon powder

¼ cup of ricotta

¼ cup of goat cheese

½ cup of Greek-style yogurt

1 ½ l ponds of fresh figs, not too ripe, quartered

Preparations:

1. Combine the cinnamon, cheeses and yogurt in a food processor, and blend until smooth.

2. Divide the mixture into different serving bowls and top each bowl with the figs, a drizzle of honey and sprinkle with walnuts. Enjoy!

Pineapple Slaw With Kale

Prep time: 15 mins

Cook time: 0 mins

Serving: 6

Ingredients:

Dressing:

1 teaspoon of   Sesame seeds toasted

1/8 teaspoon of Sriracha (optional)

1 whole lime zest

1 whole Lime juice

1 tablespoon of Honey

 1 tablespoon of Soy sauce, tamari

1 1/2 tablespoon of Peanut butter, natural

2 teaspoons Sesame oil

2 tablespoon of olive oil, extra virgin

3 teaspoons of Rice vinegar

1 teaspoons of minced Ginger root

Slaw:

1 tablespoon of toasted Sesame seeds

1 cup Edamame (soybeans), cooked

 1 cup diced Pineapple

1 cup, shredded Napa cabbage, raw

2 medium Carrots, shredded

2 cup thinly sliced Kale

Preparations:

1. To prepare the dressing: blend all the dressing ingredients together with a hand blender or food processor.

2. To prepare the slaw: combine all slaw ingredients in a medium bowl.

Toss slaw together with the dressing to coat lightly. Let stand at room temperature until ready to serve.

Almond with Macademia- Fresh Cherries

Servings: 2

Ingredients:

2 pounds of fresh cherries

1 teaspoon of stevia (or to taste)

1 tablespoon of vanilla powder

2 cups of fresh almond milk

2 ounces of almonds

10 ounces of macademia nuts

Preparation:

1. Soak almonds and Macademia nuts (best use alkaline water) for up to 12 hours.

2. When you have finished soaking, blend the nuts, vanilla powder, almond milk and Stevia together until you have a smooth and fine texture. Add more almond milk if you wish.

3. Place in the refrigerator for up to 3 hrs and serve with either grapefruit, currants or passion or fruit fresh cherries.

Alkaline Avocado Tomato Soup

Prep time: 5 mins

Cook time: 5 mins

Servings: 4

Ingredients:

A handful of fresh lovage

1 cup of alkaline water

1 fresh lemon Juice

1 garlic clove

1 small onion

1 stalk of celery

2 large tomatoes

2 small avocados, peeled and pitted

Sea salt and Parsley to taste

Preparations:

1. Cut all veggies and scoop the avocados in small pieces. Add the rest ingredients and transfer into a blender, blend until smooth. Serve chilled.

Quinoa Mango Salad With Asparagus And Nuts

Prep time: 10 mins

Cook time: 5 mins

Serving: 10

Ingredients:

1 tablespoon of Amaranth, raw

1 small chopped Apple

3/4 cup of chopped Mango

1 tablespoon of Balsamic vinegar

1 tablespoon of Olive oil

2 tablespoons of chopped Peanuts

1 cup of Muesli, with fruit and nuts

1 cup of tightly packed Baby spinach

3 minced Garlic clove

1/8 cup chopped White onion

1 cup of Asparagus

Preparations:

1. Pour 1/2 tablespoon of oil to a small pan over med-low heat and slowly sauté onion and garlic and then add in asparagus and cook until al dente but firm to the bite. Set aside.

2. Pour 1/2 tbsp of olive oil into the pan and sauté apple and mango until softens and sweetens.

3. Add cooked apple, chopped spinach, onion asparagus mix, cooked quinoa, garlic and, Italian Seasonings (optional) and muesli in a large bowl, (mix of cashews, cranberries, raisins, almonds, toasted granola and pecans) reserve few for garnish.

4. Stir in the balsamic vinegar, stir until well coated.

5. Sprinkle with reserved muesli mix and amaranth